ALIVE & WELL

Raw Food Recipes
By SUSAN PRIOR

To contact Susan or to order a copy of this book visit **alive-n-well.net**

Cover and Design by Ben Tyson
Manufactured in the United States of America

ISBN: 978-0-9864731-0-4

ACKNOWLEDGEMENTS

There are many people I must give thanks to for encouraging and supporting me along this wonderful journey:

To my friends and family (you know who you are) for listening to all my ideas and being such great food testers.

To Maggie, with much love, for being there beside me as I leapt into the unknown.

To Ben for putting this book together.

To Menlha for inviting me to the Hacienda del Sol. You have created such an amazing place. I am truly inspired every waking day.

Lastly, to my mom Virginia for understanding me more than anyone, for having confidence in me and for the guiding love along the way. I love you.

CONTENTS

SALADS & DRESSINGS

King Cabbage Salad	30
Wasabi Cucumber Salad	30
Queen Quinoa Salad	31
Sunset Salad	32
Wakame Mung Bean Salad	32
Creamy Dill Dressing	33
Dijon Dressing	33
The Hacienda Dressing	34
Hail Caesar	34
Lemon Tahini Dressing	35
Little Italy Dressing	35
Miso Ginger Dressing	36
Pine Nut Parmesan	36
Garlic Aioli Sauce	37
Sesame Sauce	37
Sweet Chili Sauce	37
Spicy Almond Sauce	38

DRINKS

Banana Avocado Shake	40
Chocolate Hemp Shake	40
Cardamom Shake	40
Mango Maca Shake	41
Mayan Cacao Shake	41
Mint Cucumber Cocktail	41
Mango Lassie	42
Monkey Madness	42
Creamsicle Smoothie	42
Spirulinade	43
Sweet Melons	43
Power Plant	43
Strawberry Fresca	44
Golden Greens	44
Green Machine	44
Almond Milk	45
Vanilla Milk	46
Chocolate Milk	46
Strawberry Milk	46
Hemp Seed Milk	46

MAINS

Beet Burgers	48
Taquitos	48
Fresh Spring Rolls	49
Quesadillas	49
Raw Falafel with Tahini Sauce	50
Wild Rice & Pecan Pilaf	51
Pizza Party	52
Rawsagna	54
Mexican Torte	55
Veggie Maki Rolls	56
Oriental Noodle Bowl	57
Veggie No Fry	58

SWEET TREATS

Banana Coconut Crepes	60
Baklava	60
Banana Toasts	61
Chocolate Mousse	61
Chocolate Brownie Cakes	62
Hemp Balls	62
Chocolate Fudge Pie	63
Coco Cacao Cream Pie	64
Dark Chocolate Ganache Tart	65
Apple Crumble	65
Macaroons	66
Ginger Cookies	66
Banana I Scream	68
Rawkie Road I Scream	68
Vanilla Bean I Scream	69
Chocolate Sauce	69
Caramel Sauce	69

INTRODUCTION

Five years ago I was introduced to raw food by a documentary film.
Soon after, I was on my way to California to study the art of raw food
preparation. I have traveled across Canada and to Costa Rica working as a
raw chef. After preparing many delicious, healing meals I decided it was time
to write a book to pass on the light from me to you.

I find that many people shy away from experimenting in the kitchen with
new techniques and recipes fearing long prep times and nasty flavours.
I am all about time management in the kitchen and I want you to know that
raw foods are very tasty and can be easy to prepare with a little forethought.
Try to incorporate a new recipe everyday made with fresh organic
ingredients. Start the morning with a big green drink or smoothie. Feel the
energy with each sip you take. Find the passion for flavourful, fresh foods.

My raw food recipes are unprocessed, whole, plant-based foods.
These foods do not reach 118ºF when heated. This is the temperature at
which nutrients are lost and enzymes destroyed. Growing up we were told
that an apple a day kept the doctor away. Imagine the benefits you'll enjoy
by incorporating fresh, organic raw foods into your diet every day! Fresh is
best. From my own experience I can assure you that once you start eating
fresh, raw foods your cravings for commercially processed, preservative-
packed foods will decrease and you will have an abundance of energy.
Try a few recipes and share them with friends and family. I'm sure they'll
tickle your taste buds and nourish your soul.

SHOPPING LIST

Having ingredients at home saves time and makes it easier to prepare raw dishes every day. Buy organic and local whenever possible with the goal of including fresh, quality ingredients in your creations. The following foods are used in my recipes and commonly in raw dishes:

Agave nectar
Apple cider vinegar
Avocado
Balsamic vinegar
Cacao butter
Cacao powder & nibs
Chia seeds
Coconut – unsweetened & shredded
Coconut oil / butter
Coconuts
Dried fruits
Evaporated cane juice
Flax oil
Flax seeds
Fresh garlic & ginger
Fruits & vegetables
Hemp seeds
Herbs & spices
Himalayan crystal salt

Honey
Irish moss
Maca powder
Maple syrup
Mesquite powder
Miso paste
Nutritional yeast
Oat groats
Olive oil
Nuts & seeds
Nut butters
Sea weeds
Sesame oil
Soy lecithin
Spirulina
Sun dried tomatoes
Tahini
Tamari sauce
Vanilla bean or extract

EQUIPMENT GUIDE

Blender Most home blenders will work just fine but a high-speed blender like a Vitamix® or Blendtec® will provide more power to process faster and much finer. All blenders will struggle trying to blend ingredients that are too dry or too thick.

Food Processor I would highly recommend the Cuisinart® Food Processor. I use it in my home daily. It is great for making pates and ice cream, slicing and grating ingredients or making dough for baking.

Coffee Grinder An electric coffee grinder can be used to grind spices, nuts, seeds, and cacao whole and nibs.

Electric Citrus Juicer This juicer makes for quick and easy juicing of all citrus fruits. If you are making fresh orange juice, or lemonade, I highly recommend one.

Juicer If you are serious about juicing and raw food, I highly recommend a Champion™ Juicer or Green Star® Juice Extractor. These juicers will extract more juice and far outlast any department store juicer. They both have attachments for grinding and milling grains, nuts and seeds. I prefer these juicers for making fruit sorbets and I Screams.

Dehydrator The Excalibur® Dehydrator works great and is used daily in my kitchen. If you want to experiment with dehydrating there are several cheaper dehydrators available at department stores that work well.

Dehydrator Sheets Non-stick, Teflon® coated sheets are used for dehydrating foods that are too sticky or too wet to put directly onto dehydrator screens.

Knives Buy the best brand of knives you can afford. Keep them sharp and dry. A good, sharp knife makes food preparation quicker and safer. You will need a chef's knife, paring knife, serrated bread knife and a cleaver (for opening coconuts).

Mandolin   The best tool for quick and easy slicing of vegetables to make veggie noodles and julienne veggies.

Micro plane / Zester   This is by far one of my favorite tools. Mincing garlic and ginger cannot be easier. This is a very sharp tool—treat it with respect.

Spiral Slicer   This is a fabulous hand-powered slicer. I use it to make noodles from vegetables. It is also great for shredding vegetables.

Nut Milk Bags   These nylon mesh bags are for straining pulp from nut milks. Paint straining bags are cheap, work well and are available at most hardware stores.

Ice Cream Scoops   All sizes work great for quick and easy portioning.

Spring Form Pans   These pans are essential for making layered pies and tortes. They enable you to serve layered dishes elegantly without sacrificing the first serving as you would scooping out of a regular pan.

KNIFE SKILLS

1. Be sure your knife is sharp.
2. When cutting be sure your fingers are curled up so that your finger nails are facing the blade.
3. Have a stable cutting surface. To prevent your cutting board from sliding around lay a damp kitchen towel underneath the cutting board.
4. Stabilize the items you're cutting by first making a flat cut that you can face toward the cutting board to prevent rolling or movement during cutting.
5. Cut with the blade's sharp edge angled slightly away from your fingers.
6. Do not use the blade to scrape or clean off your cutting surface. This will dull the blade quickly.
7. After using your knives clean them immediately by hand and dry well before storing. Wash all sharp objects individually by hand to avoid grabbing a sharp blade in a soapy sink.

PREPARATION CUTTING TECHNIQUES

Bias Cut A cut made on a 45º angle. Use this cut for attractive presentation of carrot, parsnip, celery, scallions and burdock.

Dice Cut items into small, medium or large uniform cubes. Small dice is typically pieces less than a ½ inch. Medium dice is ½ to 1 inch and large dice is greater. Uniform cuts ensure evenly cooked ingredients when cooking or steaming.

Chop Cut items into smaller pieces. When I refer to chopping the cut items will be processed after so size is not important.

Julienne Cut items into long, thin, matchstick-like pieces. This is a great cut to prepare veggies and fruits maki and spring rolls.

Mince Cut items into pieces smaller than ⅛ inch.

SOAKING & SPROUTING

It is common practice in raw food preparation to soak and/or sprout nuts, seeds and grains. Soaking removes enzyme inhibitors such as tannic acid from the grain. Once the inhibitors are washed away the grain is tastier and easier to digest. Sprouting grains makes them much easier to digest.

When soaking or sprouting use fresh, clean, filtered water in a container large enough to allow expansion of the nut, seed or grain. Glass mason jars are ideal for soaking. Cover the mouth of the jar with cheesecloth or screen and a rubber band to make rinsing and draining quick and easy. When the soaking is complete, rinse and drain the grains well in the mason jar. The grains are now ready to be used. When sprouting, soak, rinse and drain the grain several times a day for a couple of days until a sprout grows that is equal in length to the grain. If you're using a mason jar to sprout, invert the jar at an angle after draining to allow remaining moisture to flow out of the jar. Here's a chart to help you determine times for soaking and sprouting.

	SOAKING	SPROUTING (soak, rinse & drain)
Sunflower Seed Pumpkin Seed	4 hours	2 times a day for 1 to 2 days
Almond	6 hours	2 times a day for 1 to 2 days
Oat Groat Quinoa	8 hours	2 times a day for 1 to 2 days
Mung Bean	8 hours	3 times a day for 2 to 4 days
Pecan Walnut	2 hours	
Cashew Macadamia Pine Nut	1 hour	
Wild Rice	3 days — rinse & drain 2 times per day	

It is always best to use soaked or sprouted foods as soon as possible. Store them well drained in a sealed container in the refrigerator for up to 4 days. Dehydrate unused portions to be used later in other recipes.

SNACKS, STARTERS & SIDES

Corn Tortillas

Almond Cheese

Makes 1 ½ cups
Preparation time: 15 minutes

1 ½ cups soaked almonds
2 tablespoons lemon juice
1 clove minced garlic
2 teaspoons miso paste or nama shoyu
1 teaspoon salt
¼ cup chopped parsley
¼ cup water
1 small red onion finely diced

Add all ingredients, except the red onion, to a food processor and blend well. Mix in the red onion by hand or pulse lightly.

Beet Chips

Makes 3 dozen chips
Total time: 20 to 24 hours

Keeping the beets aside mix all the ingredients well in a bowl. Add the beets to the bowl and toss them until well coated. Place the beet chips on non-stick sheets without overlapping the chips.
Dehydrate at 135ºF for 1 hour, then reduce the temperature to 105ºF and continue to dehydrate for 6 to 8 more hours. Turn the beet chips over and continue to dehydrate for 8 to 12 more hours or until the chips are crispy. Once the chips have cooled store them in an airtight container in the refrigerator.

2 peeled beets sliced into thin rounds
2 tablespoons olive oil
3 tablespoons nama shoyu
1 tablespoon agave nectar
1 tablespoon nutritional yeast
1 teaspoon onion powder
1 teaspoon salt

Variations: Replace the olive oil with sesame oil. Try carrots, zucchinis, leeks, sweet potato, kale, etc., instead of beets.

Bruschetta

Serves 4 to 6
Preparation time: 20 minutes

2 cups tomatoes small diced
½ cup pitted chopped kalamata olives
2 cloves minced garlic
½ teaspoon salt
¼ cup olive oil
¼ cup crushed pine nuts
½ cup minced basil
¼ teaspoon ground black peppercorns
2 teaspoons minced red onion

Mix all the ingredients in a bowl or pulse briefly in a food processor. Serve on raw crackers or breads. This is a great, fresh starter and especially tasty with the Garlic Toasts.

Cinnamon Raisin Almond Toasts

Makes 2 dehydrator sheets
Total time: 15 to 20 hours

In a large bowl, mix all the ingredients by hand. Place 3 cups of batter between two non-stick sheets. With a rolling pin, roll out the batter evenly so it is about ¼ inch thick. Remove the top sheet and place the batter and sheet on a screen. Score the batter into desired portions. Dehydrate at 135ºF for 1 hour, reduce the temperature to 105ºF and dehydrate for 8 to 10 more hours.

6 cups almond pulp
1 cup golden flax meal
¼ cup olive oil
⅓ cup flax oil
2 tablespoons agave nectar or honey
1 tablespoon cinnamon
¼ teaspoon almond extract
1 tablespoon coconut oil
½ cup chopped raisins
1 ½ cups water
1 teaspoon salt

Flip onto a screen and remove the non-stick sheet. Dehydrate for another 8 to 10 hours or until crisp. Store in a sealed container, in the refrigerator, for 3 to 4 days or in your freezer for 1 month. Enjoy with your favourite nut butter and sliced bananas.

Corn Chips

Makes 2 dehydrator sheets
Total time: 24 hours

Add the corn, salt, water and agave to a blender and mix until smooth. Pour into a bowl and add the flaxseed and carrot. Mix well. If the mixture thickens add more water. Spread as thin and even as you can onto non-stick sheets.

12 ounces fresh or frozen corn
1 tablespoon salt
½ cup water
2 tablespoons agave nectar
1 ½ cups ground golden flaxseed
½ cup shredded carrot

Dehydrate for 1 to 2 hours at 135ºF. This is a good time to score the chips into your desired shapes and sizes. Reduce the temperature to 105ºF and continue to dehydrate for another 8 to 10 hours. Flip onto a new dehydrator screen and peel off the sheets. Continue to dehydrate for 8 to 12 hours or until super crisp.

Variation: Add chopped cilantro, green onion, lime, or chili flakes.

Corn Tortillas

Makes 8 tortillas
Total time: 9 to 12 hours

Mix all ingredients, except the flax seed, in a blender until smooth. In a large bowl mix the corn mixture and the flaxseed by hand. You may need to add water to easily spread the mixture. Spread the mixture evenly and fairly thin onto non-stick sheets. Dehydrate for 1 hour at 140ºF, reduce to 110ºF and continue to dehydrate for another 6 hours. Flip the tortillas onto a new screen and peel off the non-stick sheet. Continue to dehydrate for 2 to 4 hours until desired texture is reached. Use as wraps, sandwiches, burritos, pizza shells, or crackers.

12 ounces fresh or frozen corn
1 cup water
1 teaspoon fresh ginger
1 teaspoon cumin powder
2 tablespoons chili powder
1 teaspoon salt
1 teaspoon pepper
1 tablespoon agave nectar
2 cups ground golden flax seed

Variation: Replace cumin and chili powder with sun dried tomatoes, black olives, and sliced onion.

Exotic Mushroom Ceviche

Serves 4
Preparation time: 20 minutes

Prepare the marinated mushrooms. In a bowl mix together the olive oil, salt, and the lime juice. Toss the mushrooms in the marinade, cover and place in a refrigerator for 2 to 4 hours.

Prepare the ceviche. Add the marinated mushrooms to the remaining ingredients. Add salt and pepper to taste. Mix by hand. To serve, portion the ceviche into individual glasses, and garnish with a slice of lemon or lime. Serve with crispy corn tortilla chips.

1 cup sliced shitake mushrooms
1 cup sliced crimini mushrooms
1 cup oyster mushrooms cut into bite sized pieces
3 juiced limes
½ teaspoon salt
2 tablespoons olive oil
½ cup small diced red onion
1 small cucumber peeled
2 seeded diced tomatoes
1 clove minced garlic
1 avocado small diced
1 seeded diced chili, serrano or ancho pepper
1 juiced zested orange
¼ cup chopped cilantro
½ teaspoon oregano

Guacamole

Serves 4
Preparation time: 10 minutes

2 ripe avocados
2 tablespoons lemon juice
1 teaspoon salt
½ teaspoon pepper
1 clove minced garlic
½ teaspoon cumin
¼ cup chopped tomato
2 tablespoons minced red onion
¼ cup chopped cilantro leaves

Add avocado, lemon juice, salt, pepper, garlic and cumin to a food processor and mix until smooth. Transfer the mixture to a bowl. Add tomato, onion and cilantro and mix by hand.

Hot Nuts

Makes 2 cups
Total time: 24 hours

2 cups soaked almonds
1 tablespoon cayenne pepper
1 ½ teaspoons Himalayan
    crystal salt or sea salt
1 tablespoon onion powder
1 teaspoon garlic powder
1 teaspoon ground ginger
2 tablespoons nama shoyu or
    wheat-free tamari sauce
1 teaspoon agave nectar

Mix all the ingredients together until well-coated with the spices. Spread the nuts onto a non-stick sheet and dehydrate at 135ºF for 1 hour. Reduce the temperature to 105ºF and dehydrate for 18 to 24 hours until the nuts are dry and crispy. Try this recipe with your favourite nuts and seeds.

Macho Taco

Makes 4 cups
Preparation time: 15 minutes

This is a flavourful taco filling or substitute for refried beans. Soak the sun dried tomatoes in warm water until soft, drain and set aside the water to add as needed while processing the remaining ingredients. Add all the ingredients, except the green onion and cilantro, to a food processor and mix until fairly smooth. Add green onion and cilantro and pulse just to combine. Serve with crackers, wraps or leafy greens.

3 cups sunflower seeds
2 cups soaked sun dried tomatoes
2 tablespoons miso paste
4 teaspoons cumin powder
4 teaspoons chili powder
1 teaspoon cayenne pepper
4 tablespoons olive oil
2 tablespoons agave nectar
1 teaspoon salt
¾ cup water (from soaking)
¼ cup chopped green onion
¼ cup cilantro loosely packed

Variations: *Roll the mixture into small balls or patties and dehydrate at 115ºF for 4 to 6 hours prior to serving. This will create a crispier texture almost like baked or lightly fried.*

Nacho Cheese

Makes 1 ½ cups
Preparation time: 10 minutes

1 cup raw cashews
1 cup water
3 tablespoons nutritional yeast
½ teaspoon salt
¼ teaspoon pepper
1 teaspoon chipotle pepper powder
    or ancho chili powder

In a blender, mix all ingredients until smooth. Serve with wraps, crackers or vegetables.

Oh Onion Rings

Makes 3 dozen rings
Total time: 24 to 30 hours

3 yellow onions sliced into
    ¼ inch thick rings
⅓ cup salt
4 tablespoons lemon juice
1 cup orange juice
1 cup hemp seeds
½ cup water
1 tablespoon honey
1 clove garlic minced
1 teaspoon minced ginger
2 tablespoons nutritional yeast

Separate the onions into rings. In a bowl mix the salt, 3 tablespoons of lemon juice and enough water to cover the onion rings. Add the onion rings to the bowl of liquid and set aside for 2 hours in the refrigerator to soften. Once the onion rings have soaked, rinse them well in cold water and strain them in a colander. Lay the rings on a dry towel and allow them to sit while you prepare the batter. Add 1 tablespoon of lemon juice and the rest of the ingredients to a blender and mix until a thick batter forms. Toss the onions and the batter in a bowl until all the rings are well coated. Lay the rings on non-stick sheets without overlapping the rings. Dehydrate at 135ºF for 1 hour, reduce the temperature to 105ºF and continue to dehydrate for 6 to 8 more hours. Turn the onion rings over and continue to dehydrate for 15 to 20 more hours or until the rings are crispy. Once the rings have cooled store them in an airtight container in the refrigerator.

Onion Bread

Makes 2 dehydrator sheets or 24 pieces of bread
Total time: 20 hours

Mix all ingredients in a large bowl until well combined. Spread mixture evenly to a ¼ inch thickness on non-stick sheets. Dehydrate for 1 hour at 140ºF, reduce the temperature to 110ºF and continue to dehydrate for 8 hours. Turn over the bread, peeling off the non-stick sheet and dehydrate for 8 to 10 more hours on the dehydrator screen. The bread should be dry but still flexible.

**2 cups ground flax seed
   (brown or golden)
3 thinly sliced yellow onions
1 cup finely chopped parsley
2 cloves minced garlic
½ cup olive oil
¾ cup nama shoyu
¼ cup honey
1 ½ cups water**

Pecan Pate

Makes 2 cups
Preparation time: 15 minutes

**2 cups soaked pecans
3 tablespoons minced chives or
   green onion
1 tablespoon nama shoyu or
   wheat-free tamari sauce
1 tablespoon minced red onion
1 clove minced garlic
2 ½ tablespoons lemon juice
¼ teaspoon fresh ground
   peppercorns
½ teaspoon salt
1 pinch cayenne pepper
2 tablespoons minced fresh parsley
1 teaspoon minced fresh dill**

In a food processor, finely grind the pecans. Add the remaining ingredients and pulse just to combine. Serve with crackers, veggies, wraps or rolls.

Really Good Corn Salsa

Serves 4
Preparation time: 15 minutes

4 tomatillos small diced
1 cup seeded diced tomatoes
¼ cup diced red onion
¼ cup chopped cilantro
2 ears of corn cut from cob
1 teaspoon chili powder
1 teaspoon salt
½ teaspoon pepper
3 teaspoons agave nectar
1 teaspoon fresh lime juice

Pulse all the ingredients lightly in a food processor until combined. Refrigerate until ready to serve.

Rosemary Flax Crackers

Makes 1 dehydrator sheet
Total time: 48 hours

1 white onion chopped
2 cloves minced garlic
1 teaspoon salt
¼ cup agave nectar
1 ¼ cups ground brown flaxseed
2 tablespoons rosemary
    fresh or dried
¼ cup chopped dried cranberries
½ cup water

Mix all the ingredients together in a bowl. Add enough water to make the mixture resemble a muffin or pancake batter. Spread the batter fairly thin onto a non-stick sheet. This will make great crispy crackers and they dehydrate much faster. Sprinkle a little rosemary, onion and cranberries over the batter. Dehydrate for 1 hour at 140ºF. Score the crackers to your desired shapes and sizes. Reduce the temperature to 110ºF and dehydrate for 6 to 8 hours and then flip onto a new screen, peel off the non-stick sheet, and dehydrate for another 10 to 12 hours until crisp.

Variation: Add chopped pecans, hazelnuts, or dried apricots.

Spicy Sweet & Salty Nuts

Serves 2 cups
Total time: 24 hours

½ cup sunflower seeds
½ cup pumpkin seeds
⅓ cup cashew
⅓ cup almonds
2 teaspoons Himalayan salt
2 tablespoons lemon juice
½ teaspoon sesame oil
2 tablespoons agave nectar
¼ teaspoon cayenne pepper

Soak, rinse and drain the seeds and nuts. Mix all the ingredients together until well coated with the spices. Spread the nuts onto a non-stick sheet and dehydrate at 135ºF for 1 hour. Reduce the temperature to 105ºF and dehydrate for 18 to 24 hours until the nuts are dry and crispy.

Stuffed Mushrooms

Makes 12 mushrooms
Total time: 5 hours 40 minutes

Prepare the mushrooms. In a shallow pan add the mushrooms, nama shoyu, vinegar, 3 tablespoons of olive oil, 1 garlic clove and a ½ teaspoon of salt. Gently toss the ingredients until well coated. Marinate for a minimum of 1 hour. For the best result—marinate overnight in the refrigerator. Make the pesto stuffing. Add the rest of the ingredients to a food processor and mix until a creamy consistency is reached. You will have to stop and scrape the sides of the processor. Remove the mushrooms from the marinade. Stuff each mushroom with pesto and place on a non-stick sheet and dehydrate at 115ºF for 4 to 6 hours prior to serving.

12 medium crimini or button mushrooms, stems removed
¼ cup extra virgin olive oil
¼ cup nama shoyu or wheat-free tamari sauce
1 tablespoon rice wine vinegar
3 cloves finely minced garlic
1 ½ teaspoons Himalayan salt
1 cup soaked almonds
3 tablespoons lemon juice
½ teaspoon cumin
1 ½ cups chopped basil
1 tablespoon minced red onion
2 tablespoons pine nuts

Dolmas

Makes 25 to 30
Preparation time: 90 minutes

Begin by preparing the zucchinis. Peel them and then julienne using a mandolin. Cut the julienned pieces into ½ inch lengths to resemble rice. Place the zucchini pieces into a strainer and add 1 teaspoon of salt. Mix gently and place the strainer over a bowl to drain.

Prepare the remaining ingredients and put into a large bowl. Using your hands, lightly squeeze any excess liquid from the zucchini rice and add to the bowl. Mix gently until well combined.

Assemble the dolmas. Place a grape leaf vein side down so that the stem of the leaf is closest to you. Place a tablespoon of the filling in the centre of the grape leaf and fold over the two sides of the leaf towards the centre. Roll the leaf tightly and away from you, tucking in any protruding leaf edges in as you go. Serve with falafel and hummus.

1 jar grape leaves

3 zucchinis
1 green onion minced
1 clove garlic minced
1 teaspoon dried oregano
½ teaspoon ground black pepper
¼ teaspoon orange zest
3 tablespoons parsley minced
3 tablespoons fresh dill minced
3 tablespoons fresh lemon juice
3 tablespoons fresh orange juice
3 tablespoons olive oil
3 tablespoons dried currants or raisins
2 tablespoons chopped pine nuts
1 tablespoon agave nectar or honey
1 tablespoon pitted kalamata olives minced

Variation: *This dish is just as delicious served as a salad. Instead of wrapping with grape leaves, chop several leaves and mix them in with the rest of the ingredients.*

Garlic Toasts

Makes 15 to 20 slices
Total time: 24 hours

Mix all ingredients together in a large bowl. Add just enough water to help bind the mixture. Form into a loaf shape and cut loaf into ¼ inch slices. Place onto a dehydrator screen and dehydrate for 1 hour at 140ºF. Reduce temperature to 105ºF and continue to dehydrate for 20 to 24 hours or until toasts are crispy. Serve with bruschetta, tapenade, nut cheeses, and sliced tomatoes or break up into croutons to jazz up any salad.

4 cups ground sesame seeds
1 ½ cups whole sesame seeds
½ cup oregano dry or fresh
3 cloves minced garlic
¼ cup agave nectar
1 pinch salt

Spicy Thai Coconut Soup

Serves 4 to 6
Preparation time: 20 minutes

2 peeled chopped zucchinis
2 cups fresh coconut water
1 cup young coconut meat
1 cup peeled seeded cucumber
½ cup lemon juice
2 tablespoons grated fresh ginger
2 cloves minced garlic
1 teaspoon salt
2 tablespoons agave nectar
1 tablespoon nama shoyu
1 tablespoon curry powder
1 teaspoon cumin
½ teaspoon cinnamon
⅛ teaspoon chili flakes
1 pinch cayenne pepper

Add all the ingredients to a blender, except 6 basil leaves, the coconut oil, olive oil and avocado. Blend until smooth. Slowly add the coconut oil and olive oil while running the blender on a low speed. Continue to blend until smooth and creamy.

Garnish with fresh basil leaves and diced avocado.

12 fresh basil leaves
¼ cup coconut oil
¼ cup olive oil
1 ripe avocado diced

Tortilla Soup

Makes 6 cups
Preparation time: 30 minutes

Remove the seeds and stem from the ancho and red peppers. Soak, rinse and drain the ancho pepper and the sun-dried tomatoes. Keep the tomato water to add while blending. In a blender, mix all the ingredients, except the garnish, at high speed until smooth. Add water to desired consistency.

Top each serving with corn, avocado and minced cilantro.

1 ancho chili pepper
1 cup sun dried tomatoes
1 cup hemp seeds
3 chopped red bell peppers
6 chopped roma tomatoes
½ chopped red onion
3 cloves minced garlic
1 teaspoon chili powder
1 teaspoon cumin powder
¼ cup cilantro leaves
1 tablespoon olive oil

Garnish

1 cup fresh corn kernels
1 avocado small diced
½ cup minced fresh cilantro

Carrot Avocado Soup

Serves 2 to 4
Preparation time: 15 minutes

Add all ingredients to a blender and mix until smooth and creamy.

Variation: Replace basil with a ¼ cup of loosely packed cilantro. Add more heat with a ¼ teaspoon of chili flakes.

2 cups carrot juice
1 ripe avocado
2 teaspoons minced ginger
1 tablespoon lemon juice
1 teaspoon minced garlic
¼ teaspoon salt
¼ teaspoon cayenne pepper
¼ teaspoon Chinese 5 spice
1 tablespoon olive oil
1 teaspoon cumin
¼ cup basil leaves

Curried Corn Coconut Soup

Serves 6
Preparation time: 20 minutes

Put a ½ cup of corn aside to add to the garnish. In a blender, whirl the soup ingredients until smooth and creamy.

Top each serving with a little corn, chili flakes, cilantro leaves and pepper.

Garnish
1 ripe avocado diced
¼ teaspoon chili flakes
¼ cup chopped cilantro leaves
1 pinch ground black peppercorns

2 cups fresh corn cut from the cob
2 cups fresh young coconut meat
2 cups coconut water
½ cup fresh orange juice
1 tablespoon fresh lemon juice
1 clove minced garlic
1 tablespoon minced ginger
2 tablespoons curry powder
1 teaspoon salt
2 tablespoons agave nectar
1 teaspoon cumin
¼ teaspoon cinnamon
1 pinch cayenne pepper
1 tablespoon nama shoyu
3 tablespoons olive oil

Zucchini Hummus

Serves 6
Preparation time: 15 minutes

In a food processor, mix all ingredients until smooth and creamy.

1 peeled zucchini chopped
½ cup sesame seeds ground into flour
¼ cup tahini paste
2 cloves garlic minced
4 tablespoons lemon juice
1 teaspoon salt
¼ teaspoon ground black pepper
1 teaspoon cumin powder
1 tablespoon agave nectar or honey
1 tablespoon olive oil
1 pinch cayenne pepper

SALADS & DRESSINGS

King Cabbage Salad

Serves 6 to 8
Preparation time: 20 minutes

2 cups finely sliced purple cabbage
2 cups finely sliced green cabbage
1 cup peeled grated carrots
1 cored apple small diced
¼ cup raisins
¼ cup olive oil
¼ teaspoon ground black pepper
2 tablespoons lemon juice
2 tablespoons agave nectar or honey
1 tablespoon cider vinegar
1 clove minced garlic
½ teaspoon Dijon mustard
2 tablespoons nama shoyu

Combine the cabbage, carrots, apple and raisins in a large bowl.
Prepare the dressing. In a blender, mix the rest of the ingredients until smooth. Slowly pour a light coating of dressing over the salad and gently toss. Store extra dressing in a glass jar in the refrigerator for 3 to 5 days.

Wasabi Cucumber Salad

Serves 6
Preparation time: 25 minutes

Cut the carrot and nori sheet into pieces 1 inch long and a ¼ inch wide. Mix the nori, carrots, cucumbers and sesame seeds in a bowl. In a separate bowl prepare the dressing by whisking the remaining ingredients until well combined. Pour the dressing over the vegetables and gently toss. Serve immediately.

1 peeled carrot julienne
4 cups peeled cucumber thinly sliced
1 nori sheet
¼ cup sesame seeds
¼ cup rice vinegar
1 teaspoon wasabi powder
2 tablespoons honey or agave nectar
1 tablespoon nama shoyu
1 teaspoon minced ginger

Queen Quinoa Salad

Serves 6
Preparation time: 25 minutes

This salad is not 100% raw but very tasty.

Cook the quinoa and let it cool in a bowl. Add the cumin, salt, black pepper, cayenne and cinnamon to the bowl and mix well. Lightly steam the broccoli until the florets turn a vibrant green. Strain and rinse the broccoli in cold water to prevent further cooking.

In a large bowl, combine the parsley, cilantro, red onion, tomato, carrot, red pepper, garlic and leafy greens. Mix well. Add the seasoned quinoa, steamed broccoli, avocado, dill weed, olive oil and lemon. Gently toss the salad and serve immediately.

2 cups cooked quinoa
1 cup lightly steamed broccoli florets
1 teaspoon cumin
1 teaspoon salt
½ teaspoon ground black pepper
1 pinch cayenne pepper
⅛ teaspoon cinnamon

¼ cup minced parsley
¼ cup minced cilantro
¼ cup minced red onion
¼ cup diced tomato
¼ cup peeled diced carrot
¼ cup diced red pepper
2 cloves minced garlic
4 cups chopped leafy greens

1 ripe diced avocado
½ teaspoon minced fresh dill weed
3 tablespoons olive oil
1 juiced lemon

Sunset Salad

Serves 6
Preparation time: 20 minutes

2 cups grated carrots
2 cups grated beets
¼ cup olive oil
¼ cup cider vinegar
1 clove minced garlic
1 tablespoon minced ginger
2 tablespoons agave nectar
1 pinch salt
1 pinch pepper
¼ cup raisins
¼ cup minced green onion
8 green or red leaf lettuce
leaves chopped

Place the carrots and beets in separate bowls. Mix the oil, vinegar, garlic, ginger, agave, salt and pepper in a blender until smooth. Pour half of the dressing into each of the bowls. Gently toss each bowl. Arrange the lettuce on a serving plate and place the carrots on one half and the beets on the other. Garnish with raisins and green onions.

Variation: Add 2 cups of grated parsnips and dress evenly.

Wakame Mung Bean Salad (inspired by Menhla)

Serves 6 to 8
Preparation time: 30 minutes

Soak the wakame for 30 minutes in water, rinse and drain. Soak the mung beans for 8 to 12 hours in water, rinse and drain. Place the beans in a strainer over a bowl. Rinse and drain the beans twice a day for 2 days or until the sprout is the same size as the bean. When ready, add all the ingredients to a large bowl and gently toss.

2 cups wakame
3 cups sprouted mung beans
¼ cup sesame oil
¼ cup nama shoyu
2 tablespoons lemon juice
1 clove minced garlic
1 tablespoon grated ginger
3 tablespoons agave nectar
¼ teaspoon cayenne pepper
2 cups shredded purple cabbage
¼ cup minced green onion
¼ cup sesame seeds

Creamy Dill Dressing

Makes 1 cup
Preparation time: 10 minutes

Put all the ingredients, except the chives, in a blender and mix until smooth and creamy. Add water as needed for the desired consistency. Use the chives as a garnish to the dressing. This dressing is especially delicious when served with thinly sliced cucumbers and garnished with chives, dill sprigs and a wedge of lemon.

½ cup soaked cashews
2 tablespoons lemon juice
1 tablespoon agave nectar
½ teaspoon salt
1 teaspoon minced garlic
1 tablespoon cider vinegar
2 tablespoons minced fresh dill
½ cup water
2 tablespoons minced chives

Dijon Dressing

Makes 1 cup
Preparation time: 5 minutes

½ cup olive oil
2 tablespoons balsamic vinegar
1 teaspoon cider vinegar
⅛ cup water
¼ cup lemon juice
2 cloves garlic
2 teaspoons Dijon mustard
2 tablespoons agave nectar or honey
1 pinch salt
1 pinch pepper
1 pinch cayenne pepper

Mix all the ingredients in a blender until smooth and creamy.

The Hacienda Dressing

Makes 2 cups
Preparation time: 15 minutes

1 peeled papaya seeded & diced
2 juiced limes
¼ teaspoon chili powder
¼ cup peeled mango diced
2 teaspoons cider vinegar
3 tablespoons tahini
2 tablespoons olive oil
¼ teaspoon salt
1 pinch cayenne pepper

Put all the ingredients in a blender and mix until smooth. Chill the dressing prior to serving. Gently toss with seasonal greens and veggies or drizzle over an exotic fruit salad.

Hail Caesar

Makes 1 ¼ cups
Preparation time: 10 minutes

A perfect dressing for all greens and especially (you guessed it) romaine.

Put all the ingredients in a blender and mix until smooth. Serve with garlic toasts or break the toasts into bits for croutons. Add whole or chopped pine nuts as a salad topper.

Variation: *Substitute 1 ½ tablespoons of agave nectar or honey for the dates.*

¼ cup water
½ cup olive oil
3 cloves minced garlic
2 celery stalks
½ nori sheet torn into pieces
1 tablespoon miso paste
¼ cup lemon juice
1 teaspoon cumin powder
¼ teaspoon mustard powder
3 pitted dates
⅛ teaspoon ground black pepper
¼ teaspoon salt

Lemon Tahini Dressing

Makes 2 cups
Preparation time: 10 minutes

This is a wonderful dressing that compliments all greens and veggies.

Put all the ingredients, except the fresh herbs, in a blender and mix until smooth. Whisk the fresh herbs by hand and add to the dressing.

This dressing will keep for weeks if refrigerated in a sealed container and the fresh herbs added just prior to serving.

1 cup water
1 cup tahini
½ cup fresh lemon juice
1 clove minced garlic
1 ½ tablespoons ground cumin
1 pinch cayenne pepper
⅛ teaspoon salt
3 tablespoons minced fresh parsley or dill

Little Italy Dressing

Makes 1 cup
Preparation time: 5 minutes

1 tablespoon balsamic vinegar
¼ cup olive oil
1 tablespoon flax oil
¼ cup water
3 tablespoons lemon juice
1 tablespoon agave nectar or honey
1 teaspoon fresh oregano minced
1 teaspoon minced red onion
½ teaspoon salt
1 clove minced garlic
¼ teaspoon mustard powder

Put all the ingredients in a blender and mix until smooth. Serve with halved cherry tomatoes, thinly sliced red onion and minced basil leaves.

This dressing will keep 3 to 4 days in the refrigerator.

Miso Ginger Dressing

Makes 3 ½ cups
Preparation time: 10 minutes

A wonderful dressing for seasonal greens, a marinade for veggies and a delicious sauce for spring rolls.

Put all the ingredients, except the water, in a blender and mix until smooth. Add water to desired consistency.

Store up to 3 to 4 days in a sealed, glass container. For longer storage life add the fresh cilantro just before using.

1 cup water
2 tablespoons miso paste
2 tablespoons lemon juice
2 tablespoons orange juice
⅛ cup cider vinegar
2 tablespoons sesame oil
¼ cup olive oil
3 tablespoons fresh ginger grated
1 clove minced garlic
1 tablespoon honey
¼ cup loosely packed minced
    cilantro leaves
1 peeled chopped zucchini
1 pinch salt

Pine Nut Parmesan

Makes 1 ½ cups
Total time: 12 hours

This is a garnish for salads.

Using a food processor, pulse all the ingredients into fine crumbs. Spread the mixture onto a non-stick sheet and dehydrate at 135ºF for 1 hour.
Reduce the temperature to 110ºF and continue to dehydrate for 8 to 12 hours or until the pine nuts are dry.

1 cup pine nuts
1 teaspoon minced garlic
⅓ teaspoon salt
1 teaspoon lemon juice
2 teaspoons nutritional yeast

Garlic Aioli Sauce

Makes 1 ½ cups
Preparation time: 10 minutes

2 cups soaked cashews
1 lemon juiced
2 cloves garlic
¼ teaspoon salt
1 pinch cayenne pepper
¼ cup water

Mix all the ingredients in a blender until smooth adding the water as needed.

Store in a refrigerator for 3 to 4 days. Use as a dip for fresh veggies or a sour cream alternative for corn chips and quesadillas.

Sesame Sauce

Makes 1 cup
Preparation time: 5 minutes

Whisk all the ingredients together in a bowl. For a quick meal add zucchini noodles and julienne veggies and toss.

½ cup nama shoyu
1 ½ tablespoons rice vinegar
1 ½ tablespoons sesame oil
1 tablespoon agave nectar or honey
1 teaspoon grated ginger

Sweet Chili Sauce

Makes 1 ½ cups
Preparation time: 5 minutes

1 cup chili paste
1 ½ teaspoons nama shoyu
1 teaspoon sesame oil
1 tablespoon agave nectar
½ cup warm water

A tasty sauce for fresh spring rolls, veggie nori rolls and the Oriental Noodle Bowl. Whisk all the ingredients together in a bowl.

Variation: *Substitute the water with coconut milk.*

Spicy Almond Sauce

Makes 2 cups
Preparation time: 10 minutes

½ cup almond butter
¼ cup nama shoyu
3 tablespoons olive oil
3 tablespoons cider vinegar
3 tablespoons honey
2 cloves minced garlic
2 tablespoons minced ginger
1 cup chopped cilantro
2 teaspoons dried chili flakes
¼ to ½ cup water

In a blender, combine all ingredients until smooth adding water until the desired consistency is reached. The sauce should be thick but easy to pour. Serve with fresh spring rolls.

DRINKS

Cardamom
Shake

Banana Avocado Shake

Serves 2 to 3
Preparation time: 5 minutes

2 chopped frozen bananas
1 ripe avocado
1 young coconut (milk and meat)
2 cups water
1 teaspoon ground cinnamon
1 teaspoon maca powder
1 pinch Himalayan salt

Combine the ingredients in a blender or food processor until smooth.

Chocolate Hemp Shake

Serves 2 to 3
Preparation time: 5 minutes

Combine the ingredients in a blender or food processor until smooth.

2 chopped frozen bananas
3 cups water
4 tablespoons hemp hearts (seeds)
3 tablespoons cacao powder
1 teaspoon vanilla
1 pinch Himalayan salt

Cardamom Shake

Serves 2 to 3
Preparation time: 5 minutes

Combine the ingredients in a blender or food processor until smooth.

Variation: Substitute water or coconut water for the almond milk

2 chopped frozen bananas
1 ripe avocado
1 teaspoon ground cardamom
1 pinch fresh ground nutmeg
1 pinch ground cinnamon
1 teaspoon vanilla
1 pinch Himalayan salt
3 cups almond milk

Mango Maca Shake

Serves 2 to 3
Preparation time: 5 minutes

Combine the ingredients in a blender or food processor until smooth. For a creamier shake you can replace the water with almond milk, coconut milk, or add 3 tablespoons of hemp hearts.

2 cups chopped frozen mangos
1 tablespoon maca powder
1 ½ inches peeled fresh ginger
3 cups water
1 tablespoon agave nectar or 3 soaked dates

Mayan Cacao Shake

Serves 2 to 3
Preparation time: 5 minutes

2 chopped frozen bananas
3 tablespoons cacao powder
1 teaspoon cacao nibs (optional)
⅛ teaspoon cayenne pepper
3 tablespoons agave nectar
1 pinch Himalayan salt
3 cups almond milk

Add the ingredients to a blender or food processor and puree until smooth.

Mint Cucumber Cocktail

Serves 2 to 3
Preparation time: 5 minutes

Blend and strain the cucumbers. Add the juice to the other ingredients in a blender or food processor and puree until smooth.

3 peeled cucumbers
¼ cup fresh mint
¼ cup fresh lemon juice
3 tablespoons agave nectar
½ cup ice cubes

Mango Lassie

Serves 2 to 3
Preparation time: 5 minutes

Combine the ingredients in a blender
or a food processor until smooth.
If you're using fresh mangos then add
2 ice cubes to the recipe.

½ cup soaked cashews
2 cups coconut water
½ cup fresh young coconut meat
2 chopped frozen mangos
1 teaspoon vanilla
¼ teaspoon ground cinnamon
1 teaspoon ground cardamom
½ cup fresh orange juice
½ teaspoon grated fresh ginger

Monkey Madness

Serves 2 to 3
Preparation time: 5 minutes

Combine the ingredients in a blender or
food processor and puree until smooth.

2 chopped frozen bananas
3 tablespoons cacao powder
2 tablespoons hemp hearts
3 tablespoons agave nectar
1 teaspoon maca powder
3 cups almond milk
1 pinch Himalayan salt

Creamsicle Smoothie

Serves 6
Preparation time: 5 minutes

Peel, seed and chop a papaya and
bananas then freeze. Combine all
the ingredients in a blender until
smooth and creamy.

1 cup frozen papaya chopped
2 cups frozen bananas chopped
4 cups fresh squeezed orange juice
1 tablespoon maca powder

Spirulinade

Serves 1
Preparation time: 5 minutes

In a blender, mix all the ingredients until smooth.

1 cup water
½ cup fresh lime or lemon juice
4 ice cubes
2 tablespoons honey
1 tablespoon maca powder
1 tablespoon spirulina
1 teaspoon fresh ginger grated

Sweet Melons

Serves 2 to 3
Preparation time: 5 minutes

Combine the ingredients in a blender or food processor and puree until smooth.

2 cups chopped ripe cantaloupe
2 cups chopped watermelon
1 cup frozen cranberries
1 tablespoon ginger grated
1 tablespoon agave

Power Plant

Serves 2 to 3
Preparation time: 15 minutes

Juice the ingredients in the order listed to be certain that all the leafy greens get pushed through.

1 inch of ginger root
2 kale leaves
1 small beet
4 leaves romaine or green lettuce
1 lemon peeled
4 celery stalks
5 washed carrots

Strawberry Fresca

Serves 2
Preparation time: 5 minutes

In a blender, mix all the ingredients until smooth. For a creamier beverage add a ½ cup of frozen, sliced bananas.

2 cups freshly squeezed orange juice
1 cup fresh or frozen strawberries
2 tablespoons fresh lime juice
½ teaspoon vanilla
2 tablespoons agave nectar or honey
1 cup ice

Golden Greens

Serves 2 to 3
Preparation time: 5 minutes

3 cups apple juice or
    fresh or frozen pineapple
¼ cup cilantro sprigs
¼ cup parsley sprigs
1 juiced lemon

Combine the ingredients in a blender or food processor until smooth. This drink can be strained through a sieve or nut milk bag to remove the pulp.

Green Machine

Serves 2 to 3
Preparation time: 15 minutes

Juice ingredients in order as listed. This will assure that all the leafy greens get pushed through the juicer.

¼ cup parsley
1 peeled lemon
1 pear
4 romaine or green lettuce leaves
2 large kale leaves
2 green apples
2 whole cucumbers
4 celery stalks

Nut & Seed Milks

Any nut or seed can be used to make milk. They are a great alternative to dairy or commercially processed soy, rice and oat milks. Nut milks can stay fresh for 2 to 3 days if sealed in a glass jar and refrigerated. Freeze milks in ice cube trays and add to smoothies or frozen dessert recipes.

Almond Milk

Makes 6 cups
Preparation time: 10 minutes

2 cups soaked raw almonds
2 dates pitted and soaked
6 cups water
1 pinch salt

Add all ingredients to a blender and start mixing at a medium speed gradually increasing to high speed. Mix until smooth. Pour the milk through a strainer or nut milk bag to separate the pulp. If you're not using the milk immediately then date, label and refrigerate for 2 days or freeze. For creamier or thicker milk reduce the amount of water used.

You can save the pulp to use again in other recipes. To prepare nut pulp for use in cookie and bread recipes start by spreading the nut pulp on a non-stick sheet. Dehydrate at 135ºF for 1 hour, reduce the temperature to 105ºF and dehydrate for 8 more hours. Flip the almond pulp over and continue to dry for 8 to 12 more hours or until there is not any moisture left in the pulp. Process the dry pulp into flour using a blender, food processor or coffee grinder.

Variation: Use coconut water instead of water.

To create and enjoy these flavoured almond milks add all ingredients to a blender and mix until smooth and creamy.

Vanilla Milk

6 cups of almond milk
1 vanilla bean or 2 tablespoons vanilla extract

Chocolate Milk

6 cups of almond milk
⅓ cup cacao powder
2 tablespoons agave nectar, maple syrup or honey

Strawberry Milk

6 cups of almond milk
1 teaspoon vanilla
1 cup fresh or frozen strawberries
2 tablespoons agave nectar, maple syrup or honey

Hemp Seed Milk

Makes 5 cups
Preparation time: 10 minutes

Mix in a blender until smooth.
Straining is not required.

Variation: Substitute 3 soaked and pitted dates for the 3 tablespoons of sweetener.

1 banana
4 cups water
½ cup hemp seeds
3 tablespoons agave nectar, honey or maple syrup
1 pinch salt

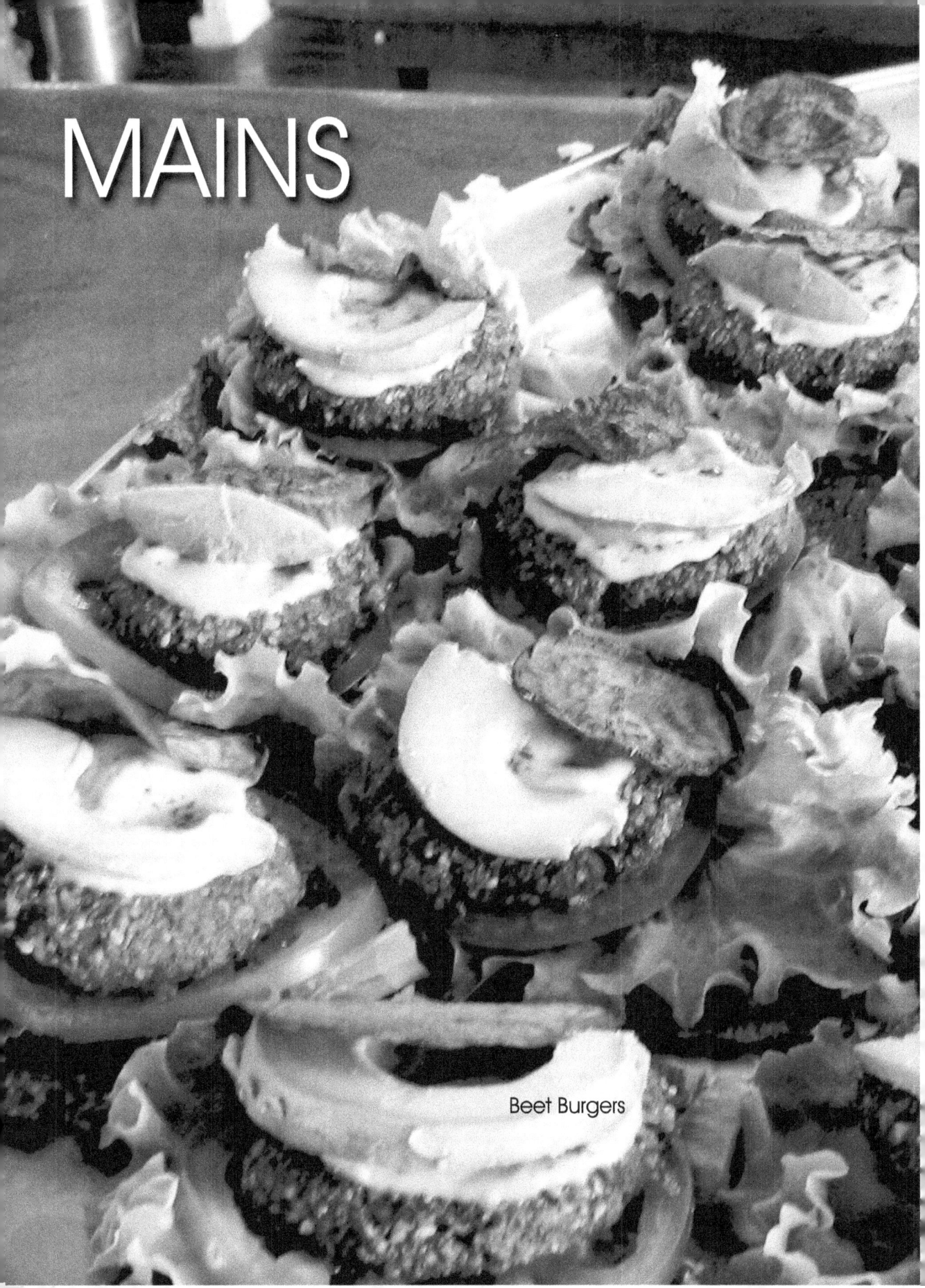

MAINS

Beet Burgers

Beet Burgers

Makes 10 to 15 patties
Preparation time: 40 minutes

In a food processor, blend all the ingredients until they resemble chili or ground beef. Transfer into a large bowl and mix. With a large ice cream scoop, or spoon, scoop out a ¼ to ½ cup and form into patties. This recipe is ready to eat! Serve burrito-style wrapped in your choice of tortilla or leafy greens or like a burger placing the patty between 2 pieces of Onion Bread. Top the patties with any of the following: sliced avocado, tomato, thinly sliced red onion, sprouts, lettuce, marinated and dehydrated mushrooms or almond cheese. For a crispier, grilled texture place the patties on a dehydrator screen and dehydrate at 145ºF for 1 hour. Reduce the temperature to 105ºF and continue to dehydrate for 2 to 4 more hours.

1 ½ cups soaked almonds
½ cup soaked sunflower seeds
¾ cups ground brown flaxseed
¾ cups soaked raisins
2 celery stalks medium diced
2 peeled carrots medium diced
½ cup peeled grated beet
⅓ cup finely diced red onion
¾ cup zucchini medium diced
1 clove minced garlic
2 tablespoons lemon juice
1 tablespoons Himalayan salt
2 tablespoons miso paste
2 teaspoons black sesame seeds

Taquitos

Serves 6 to 8
Preparation time: 30 minutes

Begin by preparing the recipes listed. Cut each tortilla square in half to make rectangles. Spread the Macho Taco on half of the tortilla along its longest edge. On top of that spread the Nacho Cheese. Roll up the longest edge tightly and serve with salsa and Guacamole.

Nacho Cheese
Really Good Corn Salsa
Macho Taco
Guacamole
Corn Tortillas

Fresh Spring Rolls

Serves 4 to 6
Preparation time: 45 minutes

Begin by preparing a batch of sauce. Thinly julienne the red pepper, carrot, mango and cucumber. Once the fillings and sauce are ready begin assembly of the rolls. Add 2 cups of warm water to a shallow baking dish or pie plate. Place a rice paper into the water and soak until it is pliable. Place the softened rice paper on a flat working surface and pat dry with a clean towel. Place a fresh leaf of lettuce on the rice paper then 2 tablespoons of sauce in the middle of the lettuce. Add a few pieces of each filling, fold in the ends of the rice paper and roll. Serve cut in half with a side bowl of extra sauce.

1 batch of Sweet Chili Sauce or Spicy Almond Sauce
8 rice paper wraps
1 red pepper
1 peeled carrot
1 peeled mango
1 peeled seeded cucumber
2 cups pea shoots or sunflower sprouts
8 green leaf lettuce leaves
2 thinly sliced avocados
1 cup cilantro leaves

Quesadillas

Serves 8
Total time: 9 hours

Prepare the recipes listed. To assemble the quesadillas, place the corn tortillas onto 2 dehydrator screens. Spread the Macho Taco on to half the tortilla and on the other half spread the Nacho Cheese. Fold in half to make triangles. Dehydrate at 110ºF for 1 to 2 hours prior to serving. Serve with a side of Guacamole and salsa.

Nacho Cheese
Really Good Corn Salsa
Macho Taco
Guacamole
Corn Tortillas

Variation: Substitute Corn Tortillas with large leafy greens and roll like a burrito. Try Almond Cheese or Pecan Pate and fresh veggies for the filling.

Raw Falafel with Tahini Sauce

Makes 15 to 20 falafel balls
Preparation time: 30 minutes

Process the falafel ingredients in a food processor until smooth or to desired texture. Roll the mixture into balls or press into small patties. A small ice cream scoop works like a charm. The falafel is ready to serve. For a crispier texture (like pan-fry) dehydrate at 110ºF for a few hours prior to serving.

Prepare the tahini sauce. Slowly add water while mixing the tahini, olive oil, lemon juice, garlic and salt in a blender until the desired consistency is reached.

Wrap falafel in your choice of leafy greens. Garnish with red onion, tomatoes, parsley and tahini sauce.

Falafel

2 cups soaked raw almonds
¼ cup ground sesame seeds
¼ cup tahini
1 juiced lemon
1 clove garlic
2 teaspoons ground cumin
1 teaspoon salt
1 cup minced cilantro
fresh ground peppercorns
**   to taste**

Tahini Sauce

¼ cup tahini
¼ cup olive oil
⅛ cup lemon juice
¼ cup water
2 cloves garlic
1 teaspoon sea salt

fresh leafy greens for wrapping
½ cup diced red onion
½ cup diced tomatoes
¼ cup minced parsley

Wild Rice & Pecan Pilaf

Serves 6
Preparation Time: 3 hours 30 minutes

If you have a dehydrator, begin by blooming your wild rice in a shallow glass dish. Cover the rice with water and put the dish in the dehydrator for 18 to 24 hours at 120ºF. After 10 hours have passed, drain and rinse the rice then cover again with fresh water and continue dehydrating. The rice is ready when the husk has cracked and opened exposing the soft centre.

If you don't have a dehydrator, begin by soaking the wild rice for 3 days.

Prepare the marinade. In a blender, mix the ingredients until well combined.

In a glass baking dish, add the carrot, red pepper, mushrooms, broccoli and marinade. Mix by hand. Place the dish inside a dehydrator for 3 hours at 110ºF. In a bowl, combine the wild rice and dehydrated ingredients. Mix in the chopped pecans and cranberries by hand. Garnish with the minced parsley.

2 cups wild rice soaked
1 peeled carrot small diced
1 red pepper small diced
1 cup crimini or button mushrooms sliced thin
1 cup broccoli cut into small florets
½ cup chopped pecans
¼ cup dried cranberries
2 tablespoons minced Italian parsley

Marinade

¼ cup nama shoyu or wheat-free tamari sauce
2 teaspoons fresh lemon juice
2 teaspoons onion powder
1 clove minced garlic
2 tablespoons olive oil
2 tablespoons agave nectar or honey
1 pinch cayenne pepper

Pizza Party

Makes 2 dehydrator sheets
Total time: 24 hours

Pizza Crust

In a large bowl, combine the flax and chia seeds and set aside. In a blender, mix 1 cup of water and the remaining ingredients until smooth. Pour the blended mixture into the dry seeds and mix well. Add just enough water to make the dough easy to spread. Spread the dough evenly a ¼ inch thick onto non-stick sheets. Score the dough into desired servings prior to dehydrating. For individual pizzas place a cup of dough onto the sheet, spread into a 6 inch round and repeat. Dehydrate at 140ºF for 1 hour, reduce the temperature to 105ºF and dehydrate for 8 to 10 more hours. Flip the dough onto dehydrator screen and continue to dehydrate for 8 to 10 hours or until crisp.

2 cups water (add as needed)
1 cup ground golden flax seeds
1 cup ground chia seeds
¼ cup flax oil
¼ cup olive oil
3 cloves minced garlic
¼ cup fresh lemon juice
¼ cup agave nectar or honey
¼ cup chopped yellow onion
¼ cup soaked sun dried tomatoes
2 tablespoons dried Italian seasoning
¼ cup chopped fresh oregano or basil
2 tablespoons nutritional yeast

Choose one of the following pizza flavours to prepare the toppings.

Greek

Prepare a batch of Almond Pesto Cheese. Spread the pesto cheese on the pizza crusts then add the toppings in the order listed.

Almond Pesto Cheese
1 cup sliced cherry tomatoes
2 tablespoons minced basil leaves
¼ cup chopped kalamata olives
½ red onion thinly sliced
¼ cup chopped pine nuts
1 cup fresh sprouts or baby greens

Aloha

Prepare a batch of Almond Cheese. Mix the pineapple, red pepper, red onion, salt and nama shoyu. Dehydrate in a glass baking dish at 110ºF for 3 hours. Once ready, spread the Almond Cheese on the pizza crust and add the dehydrated toppings followed by the avocado, tomatoes and sprouts.

Almond Cheese
1 cup pineapple small diced
1 thinly sliced red pepper
½ cup thinly sliced red onion
1 pinch salt
1 tablespoon nama shoyu
1 avocado small diced
½ cup sliced cherry tomatoes
1 cup fresh sprouts or baby greens

Marinara

Prepare a batch of Almond Cheese, Bruschetta and Marinara Sauce. Mix the mushrooms, olive oil, nama shoyu, lemon juice and salt in a glass, baking dish. Put the dish in a dehydrator at 110ºF for 3 hours. Once ready, spread the Almond Cheese on the pizza crust and then the Marinara sauce and add the dehydrated toppings followed by the Brushcetta, pine nuts and sprouts.

Almond Cheese
Bruschetta
Marinara Sauce
4 cups thinly sliced crimini mushrooms
2 tablespoons olive oil
1 tablespoon nama shoyu
2 tablespoons lemon juice
¼ teaspoon salt
¼ cup chopped pine nuts
1 cup fresh sprouts or baby greens

Rawsagna

Makes one 9 inch baking dish and serves 4
Preparation time: 3 hours

To make this raw lasagna prepare the following elements and then assemble.

Marinated Mushrooms & Broccoli

In a shallow pan, toss all the ingredients until the veggies are well coated. Dehydrate at 110ºF for 2 to 3 hours or refrigerate for 3 to 4 hours before assembling.

2 cups thinly sliced mushrooms
1 head broccoli cut into small florets
1 teaspoon cumin
1 teaspoon salt
½ teaspoon black pepper
2 tablespoons tamari or soy sauce
2 tablespoons olive oil

Almond Pesto Cheese

Add ingredients to a food processor and mix to a creamy consistency resembling ricotta cheese. Put in a bowl and set aside.

2 cups soaked almonds
¼ cup lemon juice
2 cloves minced garlic
1 teaspoon salt
1 ½ cups chopped basil
1 tablespoon olive oil
2 tablespoons minced red onion

Marinara Sauce

Soak the sun dried tomatoes and save the drained water.

In a food processor, mix all the ingredients well. If the sauce is too thick add the tomato water to the desired consistency.

5 seeded chopped tomatoes
2 seeded chopped red peppers
¼ cup diced red onion
2 cloves minced garlic
1 cup soaked sun dried tomatoes
1 tablespoon lemon juice
1 teaspoon cumin
1 teaspoon salt
½ teaspoon black pepper
⅛ teaspoon cayenne pepper
1 tablespoon honey

Rawsagna Noodles

Slice zucchinis lengthwise as thin as possible, using a mandolin or peeler, to make noodles.

3 large zucchinis
2 cups chopped spinach
2 cups sunflower sprouts
    or pea-shoots

Assembly of the Rawsagna

Use a 9 inch spring form pan. Start each of the following layers with a layer of zucchini noodles:

1. Spread a ¼ cup of Marinara with ½ a cup of the spinach.
2. Spread a ¼ cup of Almond Pesto cheese and then one half of the Marinated Mushrooms and Broccoli.
3. Repeat layers 1 and 2.
4. Repeat layer 1.
5. Top with Almond Pesto Cheese and sunflower sprouts.

Mexican Torte

Serves 4
Preparation time: 90 minutes

Prior to assembling this 12 layered festive dish you will need to prepare the recipes listed. Use a mandolin to slice the zucchinis lengthwise. In a 9 inch spring form pan, start each of the following layers with a layer of zucchini noodles:

Nacho Cheese
Really Good Corn Salsa
Macho Taco
Guacamole
6 peeled sliced zucchinis
2 cups baby spinach
2 cups sunflower sprouts

1. Spread Macho Taco over the zucchini.
2. Pour and spread some Nacho Cheese covering it with a layer of spinach.
3. Spread some Corn Salsa over the zucchini.
4. Spread Guacamole over the zucchini.
5. Spread Macho Taco over the zucchini layer and add some more Nacho Cheese.
6. Add Corn Salsa and sunflower sprouts.

Let this torte set in the refrigerator for 1 to 2 hours before serving.

Veggie Maki Rolls

Serves 6 to 8
Preparation time: 60 minutes

Set aside the nori sheets until you're ready to roll. Juice 8 to 10 carrots to create 2 cups of pulp. Enjoy the juice while you create this dish. Add the carrot pate ingredients to a large bowl and mix well. The pate is taking place of the sushi rice that is usually used in maki rolls.

Prepare the veggie fillings. Julienne the red pepper, cucumber, mango and avocado and set aside.

In a blender, mix the secret sauce until super smooth and set aside a ¼ cup for garnish.

Veggie Filling

1 red pepper
½ cucumber peeled seeded
1 ripe peeled mango
1 ripe avocado
2 cups pea shoots or sunflower sprouts
½ cup cilantro leaves
¼ cup sesame seeds

8 nori sheets

Carrot Pate

2 cups carrot pulp
2 finely minced celery stalks
1 tablespoon finely minced
    red onion
1 teaspoon grated ginger
1 ½ teaspoons cumin
1 teaspoon ground black
    peppercorns
½ teaspoon salt
2 tablespoons finely
    chopped dulse
1 pinch of cayenne pepper

Susan's Secret Sauce

½ cup tahini
½ cup lemon juice
½ cup water
¼ cup olive oil
¼ teaspoon sesame oil
1 ½ teaspoons agave nectar

Get ready to roll. Place a nori sheet on a bamboo rolling mat shiny side facing down. Smear 4 to 5 tablespoons of the carrot pate evenly across the bottom half of the nori sheet leaving a 1 inch strip of the sheet clear along the edge closest to you. Next, place a portion of sliced veggies lengthwise across the pate. It's a nice touch to place some of the veggies so that they extend a ½ inch over the ends of the nori sheet. Curl the bottom of the nori up and over the vegetables. Tuck the nori under a little, and bring the mat up over the roll.

Continue to roll gripping tightly to ensure the roll is not loose and pull the mat back before it tucks into the roll. Wet the edges of the nori with a little water to help keep the roll together. Use a serrated knife to cut the roll. Start in the middle and cut the roll into 1 inch pieces at a slight angle. Serve with a side of the secret sauce.

Variations: Use any sliced or shredded veggies to roll into the maki rolls. Parsnip, jicama, spinach, oranges, mushrooms, green onions, etc...be creative. Serve with a side of nama shoyu, wasabi and some pickled ginger.

Oriental Noodle Bowl

Serves 4 to 6
Preparation time: 25 minutes

To make the sauce mix all the ingredients in a blender until smooth.

Use a mandolin to julienne the zucchini or a spiral slicer to make zucchini noodles. Lightly salt the zucchini noodles. The salt will draw out moisture so store the noodles in a strainer over a bowl in the refrigerator prior to serving. Put all the noodle ingredients in a large bowl. Add just enough of the sauce to the bowl to coat the vegetables and gently toss. Store extra sauce in the refrigerator.

Garnish each serving with some hemp seeds.

Sauce

¼ cup hemp seeds or
    white sesame seeds
¼ cup water
2 tablespoons nama shoyu
2 tablespoons rice wine vinegar
3 tablespoons agave nectar
1 tablespoon minced fresh ginger
1 tablespoon miso paste
2 tablespoons olive oil
1 teaspoon sesame oil
1 teaspoon Chinese 5 spice powder

Noodles

5 peeled zucchinis
2 seeded red peppers diced
½ cup chopped cilantro leaves
3 green onions cut on the bias

Veggie No Fry

Serves 6
Total time: 4 hours

Start by preparing the veggies.
Cut the broccoli and cauliflower into small florets. Slice the carrots and celery thin on a diagonal. Slice the mushrooms a ¼ inch thick.

In a large bowl, whisk the marinade thoroughly. Add all the veggies, except the zucchini noodles, to the marinade and toss until well coated.
Transfer the marinated veggies into 2 shallow baking dishes and place in the dehydrator for 4 hours at 115ºF.
After the veggies have been dehydrating for about 2 hours give them a quick stir.

Using a mandolin, or spiral slicer, julienne the zucchini. Salt the zucchini noodles and toss gently. The salt will draw out moisture so store the noodles in a strainer over a bowl in the refrigerator prior to serving.

Serve the dehydrated veggies over the zucchini noodles.

The Veggies

2 cups fresh pineapple diced
2 bell peppers julienne
1 head broccoli
1 head cauliflower
4 peeled carrots
2 celery stalks
3 ears of corn cut off the cob
2 medium red onions diced
3 cloves minced garlic
2 cups crimini or button mushrooms sliced

Marinade

½ cup nama shoyu or wheat-free tamari sauce
¼ cup sesame oil
2 tablespoons honey or agave nectar
2 tablespoons lemon juice
½ teaspoon black pepper
2 teaspoons fresh ginger grated

Zucchini Noodles

3 zucchinis peeled
½ teaspoon salt

SWEET TREATS

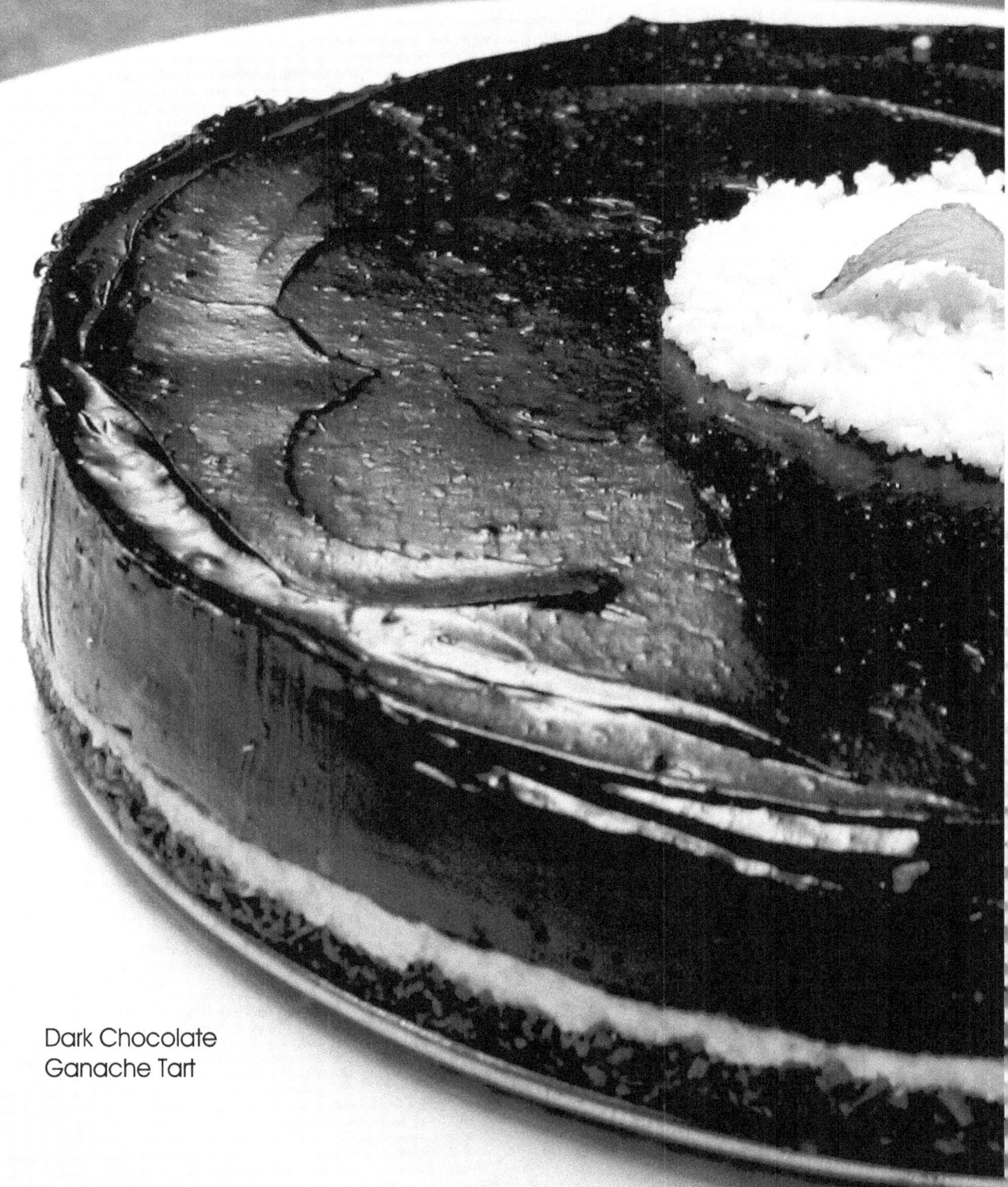

Dark Chocolate
Ganache Tart

Banana Coconut Crepes

Makes 8 to 10 six inch crepes
Total time: 12 hours

Put the flax into a bowl. In a blender, mix all the other ingredients until smooth and creamy. Pour the blended ingredients into the flax and stir until well combined. You may need to add a little water if the batter is too thick. Spread the batter onto non-stick sheets an ⅛ inch thick and into 6 inch rounds or you can spread evenly across the whole sheet and cut into shapes. Dehydrate at 140ºF for 1 hour, reduce the temperature to 105ºF and continue to dehydrate for 3 to 4 more hours. Flip the crepes onto a dehydrator screen and dehydrate for another 3 to 4 hours. The crepes should be flexible enough to fold over a filling without cracking. Once ready spread your favourite butter or sliced fruits over the crepe. Fold into a ½ circle and cut into 3 pie-shaped servings. Garnish with shredded coconut, sliced bananas and chocolate sauce.

1 cup ground golden flaxseed
2 ripe bananas
2 cups fresh young coconut meat
1 ½ cups coconut water
1 teaspoon vanilla
½ teaspoon cinnamon powder
1 tablespoon maple syrup or agave nectar
1 pinch of salt

Variation: Add a ⅓ cup of cacao powder for chocolate banana coconut crepes.

Baklava

Serves 4 to 6
Preparation time: 20 minutes

Use a 9 inch baking dish or make individual servings. Use a mandolin to slice the apples thin. Process the nuts to crumbs. Mix the nuts with the agave nectar and spread over each apple layer. Make at least 3 layers. Press the layers down so they are fairly compact. Top with more nuts and agave. Serve and enjoy.
This dessert is equally tasty with walnuts or almonds instead of pistachios.

4 apples sliced paper thin
4 cups pistachios
8 tablespoons agave nectar

Banana Toasts

Makes 1 dehydrator sheet
Total time: 20 to 24 hours

In a bowl mix the almond pulp, ground flax and walnuts and set aside. In a food processor, blend the banana and dates until they are creamy. Add the rest of the wet ingredients and salt and mix until creamy. Add the wet ingredients to the dry and mix well. Once mixed, form the mixture into a small loaf shape approximately 10 inches long and 2½ inches high. I like to cover the top of the loaf with hemp seeds. Slice the loaf with a serrated knife into ¼ inch slices. Thicker slices will take longer to dehydrate. Dehydrate at 135ºF for 1 hour, then reduce the temperature to 105ºF and continue to dehydrate for 15 to 20 hours or until crisp. The batter can be made into cookies, crackers or any shape you can imagine. This recipe will last in the refrigerator for 4 to 5 days, and can be stored in an airtight container in the freezer for a month.

2 cups almond pulp*
¾ cup ground golden flax
½ cup chopped walnuts
2 ripe bananas
4 pitted dates
1 teaspoon vanilla
1 tablespoon raw almond butter
2 tablespoons agave or honey
¼ cup flax oil
2 tablespoons olive oil
1 cup water
2 tablespoons coconut oil
1 teaspoon salt (to taste)

From making nut milk. Substitute almonds ground into flour.

Chocolate Mousse

Serves 6
Preparation time: 10 minutes

Mix in a food processor until smooth.

3 ripe avocados
1 ½ cup cacao powder
1 ¼ cup honey
1 tablespoon vanilla
2 teaspoons coconut oil
½ teaspoon salt
1 teaspoon cinnamon

Chocolate Brownie Cakes

Serves 8
Total time: 2 hours

In a food processor mix 1 cup of the walnuts with the dates until they form a fine crumb consistency. Add the rest of ingredients and process until thoroughly combined. Add just enough date water to ensure the ingredients bind together.
Mix a ¼ cup of chopped walnuts by hand into the mixture. Divide the mixture into small muffin tins or spread evenly into a glass baking dish and chill for 2 hours. Serve with Banana I Scream and Chocolate Sauce.

1 ¼ cup walnuts
¼ cup water (from the dates)
12 pitted soaked dates or
**   1 cup soaked raisins**
⅓ cup cacao powder
1 teaspoon vanilla
1 teaspoon mesquite powder
1 pinch of salt

Hemp Balls

Makes 30 to 40 balls
Preparation time: 1 hour

Use a food processor to turn the dates into a paste. Add some of the date water to make a creamy paste. Add the cashews, salt and coconut oil. Process until a consistency similar to smooth peanut butter is reached.
Put the mixture into the freezer for 30 minutes.   The balls are easier to form when the mixture is firm. Form the mixture into 1 inch balls and roll in hemp seeds.

20 pitted soaked dates
**   (save the water)**
2 cups ground dry cashews
1 pinch of salt
¼ cup coconut oil
½ cup shelled hemp seeds

Variation: Dip the balls into raw cacao powder, shredded coconut, crushed nuts or agave nectar prior to rolling in hemp seeds.

Chocolate Fudge Pie

Serves 10 to 12
Total time: 3 hours

This pie is made in layers. Start with the crust. In a bowl, combine ground walnuts, coconut flour, and cocoa powder. In a food processor, process the remaining crust ingredients until smooth. Mix the wet ingredients into the dry ingredients.
Press the crust mixture evenly into the bottom of a 9 inch spring form pan, then place the pan in the freezer until the next layer is ready.

In a food processor, combine the centre layer ingredients until smooth and creamy. Pour the mixture over the crust, and evenly spread. Put the pan back in the freezer until the top layer is ready.

Process the top layer ingredients until smooth and creamy. Add to the top of the pie and spread evenly. Freeze the pie for 2 to 3 hours to allow it to set before cutting. Serve with chocolate sauce or fresh strawberries.

Crust

4 cups walnuts*
2 cups coconut flour**
¼ cup cacao powder
1 cored chopped apple
12 pitted soaked dates
3 tablespoons coconut oil
¼ teaspoon salt

Centre Layer

3 ½ cups soaked cashews
¼ cacao powder
¾ cup agave nectar

Top Layer

2 ripe avocados
3 tablespoons cacao powder
¾ cup agave

  * *Process into fine crumbs.*
** *Process shredded coconut into flour.*

Coco Cacao Cream Pie

Serves 8 to 12
Preparation time: 3 hours

Make this tasty pie in layers starting with the crust. In a food processor, mix the crust ingredients to a crumb consistency. Be careful to not over process or the crust will be too doughy. Press the crust into a 9 inch spring form pan or pie plate and place in the freezer until the filling is ready.

Prepare the coconut cream layer. Soak the raisins for 15 minutes and drain well. In a blender, mix the coconut milk & meat, raisins, vanilla and salt until smooth. Add the lecithin and coconut oil and continue blending until the mixture is creamy. Take the crust out of the freezer and pour the filling evenly over it. Put the pie back in the freezer for about 1 hour to set.

Prepare the cacao layer. In a blender, mix the Irish moss with a ½ cup of the almond milk until smooth. To this add all ingredients except the lecithin and coconut oil. Blend until smooth then add the lecithin and coconut oil and continue blending until the mixture is smooth. Take the pie out of the freezer and pour the mixture over the firm coconut cream layer. Place the pie back in the freezer to set for 1 hour. Top with a thin layer of coconut flakes or drizzle some chocolate sauce. Each of these layers makes a great pie on its own; double the quantities for a full pie.

Crust

1 teaspoon coconut oil
2 ½ cups dried coconut
¼ teaspoon vanilla
⅛ teaspoon salt
¼ cup raisins

Coconut Cream

1 ¼ cups fresh coconut milk
1 cup fresh young coconut meat
¾ cup soaked raisins
½ teaspoon vanilla
⅛ teaspoon Himalayan salt
3 tablespoons lecithin
½ cup coconut oil

Cacao

½ ounce Irish moss
1 ½ cups almond milk
¼ cup soaked raisins
¼ cup honey or agave nectar
2 tablespoons vanilla
⅛ teaspoon Himalayan Salt
⅓ cup cacao powder
1 tablespoon lecithin
½ cup coconut oil

Dark Chocolate Ganache Tart

Makes one 9 inch tart
Total time: 3 hours and 30 minutes

Start by making the crust for the tart. In a food processor, mix the walnuts, cane sugar, coconut oil and a ½ cup of cacao powder to form a fine, crumbly dough. Spread evenly in the bottom of a 9 inch spring form pan. Place the pan in the refrigerator until the ganache filling is ready. In a food processor or high-speed blender, blend the rest of the cacao and the maple syrup until smooth. Add the coconut butter and lecithin and continue to process until smooth.

1 cup ground walnuts
¼ cup evaporated cane sugar
¼ cup warmed coconut oil
2 ¾ cups cacao powder
2 ¼ cups maple syrup
¾ cup coconut butter
1 teaspoon lecithin

Variation: Add a layer of Mint Cream.
1 ½ cups coconut meat
2 tablespoons cacao butter, melted
2 tablespoons agave
1 teaspoon mint extract
Blend all ingredients until creamy.

Taste the ganache to make sure it is not grainy. Pour into the chilled tart crust. Lightly lift and drop the pan on the counter to release any air bubbles. Place the pan in the refrigerator to set for at least 3 hours.

Apple Crumble

Serves 4 to 6
Preparation time: 15 minutes

Begin by making the crumble. Process the walnuts into a rough crumb. Mix in a ¼ cup of agave and salt by hand. I like to dehydrate the crumble for a few hours at 110ºF to give it that baked texture. In a food processor, puree the apples until they resemble a thick sauce.

2 cups walnuts
¼ teaspoon salt
5 cored apples
¾ cup of agave nectar or honey
1 ½ teaspoons cinnamon
1 pinch of nutmeg

Add the cinnamon, nutmeg, agave and mix. Spoon the apple mixture into dessert dishes and top with the crumble. Serve with a scoop of I Scream.

Macaroons

Makes 40 macaroons
Total time: 20 to 24 hours

In a bowl, mix everything together and form into small balls. Dehydrate at 135ºF for 1 hour, reduce the temperature to 110ºF and continue to dehydrate for 20 to 24 hours on a dehydrator screen.

3 cups dried unsweetened coconut
1 ½ cups cacao powder
1 cup agave nectar or honey
⅓ cup coconut oil
1 tablespoon vanilla
½ teaspoon salt
2 tablespoons maca powder

Variations: *For vanilla macaroons replace cacao powder with almond flour, add chopped cranberries, or dried pineapple. For a chocolate cherry macaroon add chopped dried cherries to the macaroon recipe.*

Ginger Cookies

Makes about 2 dozen cookies
Preparation time: 20 minutes

In a food processor, mix all ingredients until smooth. Add small amounts of water to make cookie dough. On a non-stick sheet, evenly spread the dough a ¼ inch thick. Score the dough to make the desired cookie shapes prior to dehydrating. Dehydrate at 110ºF for 8 to 12 hours. Flip onto a new screen, peel off the non-stick sheet and continue dehydrating for 8 to 12 more hours.

2 cups soaked almonds
1 cup soaked dates
2 teaspoons lemon juice
2 tablespoons minced ginger
1 ½ tablespoons molasses
1 tablespoon cinnamon
1 tablespoon honey
½ teaspoon nutmeg
⅛ teaspoon ground cloves
¼ teaspoon salt

Variations: *Use cookies in an ice cream sandwich. For a chocolate cookie, replace the ginger with a ½ cup of cacao powder and 2 tablespoons of vanilla.*

Three Little Cookies

Makes 48 cookies
Preparation time: 20 minutes

This is a great cookie recipe that can be varied into many different flavors. Here is the basic recipe followed by a couple of variations. Be creative and play around adding your favorite cookie ingredients.

Soak the oat groats over night in 2 to 3 cups of fresh water. Drain and rinse. In a food processor, process the oat groats, half the raisins and the rest of the ingredients until it has a smooth consistency. Mix in the remaining raisins by hand. Form into cookies or balls. Freeze for 1 hour and serve. For a crispier texture place the dough onto non-stick sheets and press down to form flat cookies. Dehydrate at 135ºF for 1 hour, reduce the temperature to 110ºF and continue dehydrating for 8 more hours. Flip the cookies over on to a dehydrator screen and continue to dry for 4 more hours. These can be served with a nice moist center or you can dehydrate longer for crisp cookies.

1 cup oat groats
½ cup nut butter
½ cup soaked raisins
3 tablespoons agave nectar or honey
½ teaspoon vanilla
¼ teaspoon salt
1 teaspoon cinnamon
1 tablespoon coconut or olive oil

Tropicana Bites

Add to the Basic Cookie recipe:
½ cup dried coconut
¼ cup finely chopped dried pineapple
½ teaspoon orange zest
2 teaspoons coconut butter

Chocolate Chippers

Add to the Basic Cookie recipe:
¼ cup organic cacao powder
1 tablespoon chopped cacao nibs
1 tablespoon coconut butter
1 tablespoon mesquite powder (for a caramel kick)

Banana I Scream

Serves 4 to 6
Preparation time: 1 hour

8 frozen bananas
1 teaspoon vanilla extract or 1 vanilla bean pod cut and pulp removed

This can be made with a Champion™ Juicer, a food processor or a high-speed blender. To use a processor or blender, first slice the bananas into rounds and freeze. Add the frozen bananas and vanilla to a blender and mix until smooth and creamy.   You will have to stop and scrape down the container to ensure the bananas are processed completely. Place the mixture into a shallow dish and freeze for 1 hour prior to serving.

To use a Champion™ Juicer with the blank insert, first slice the bananas into halves and freeze. Feed the frozen bananas into the juicer. Mix the vanilla and the pureed bananas in a dish and freeze for 1 hour. Scoop and serve.

Rawkie Road I Scream

Serves 4
Preparation time: 1 hour 30 minutes

Soak the cashews for 1 hour, rinse and drain. To a blender, add the cashews, cacao powder, coconut oil, sweetener, vanilla, almond milk, lecithin and salt; mix until smooth and creamy. Add the rest of the ingredients to the blended mixture. Blend on a medium speed briefly. Place in the freezer to set for 1 hour. Enjoy.

2 cups soaked cashews
⅓ cup cacao powder
½ cup coconut oil or butter
¼ cup agave nectar or maple syrup
1 tablespoon vanilla
1 cup almond milk
1 teaspoon lecithin
1 pinch salt
¼ cup almond butter
¼ cup chopped pecans
¼ cup hemp seeds
1 tablespoon cacao nibs

Vanilla Bean I Scream

Serves 4 to 6
Preparation time: 1 hour 30 minutes

Scrape the inside of the vanilla bean and discard the outer shell. Put all the ingredients in a blender and blend until smooth and creamy. Place the mixture into the freezer to set for 1 hour then serve.

2 cups soaked cashews
¼ cup coconut oil or butter
⅓ cup agave nectar
1 vanilla bean
1 ½ cups almond milk or hemp milk
1 teaspoon lecithin

Chocolate Sauce

Makes 1 ½ cups
Preparation time: 5 minutes

¼ cup water
½ cup cacao powder
1 cup agave nectar or maple syrup
1 tablespoon vanilla
1 pinch salt

Mix in a blender until smooth.

Caramel Sauce

Makes 1 ½ cups
Preparation time: 10 minutes

Soak the nuts for 1 hour, rinse and drain. Put all the ingredients in a blender, pulse and then gradually increase the speed until the sauce is smooth and creamy. For a thinner consistency add more almond milk. Serve over Baklava or Banana I Scream.

1 cup soaked cashews or
    macadamia nuts
¼ cup almond milk
½ cup agave nectar or honey
½ teaspoon vanilla
2 teaspoons mesquite powder
½ teaspoon salt

www.ingramcontent.com/pod-product-compliance
Lightning Source LLC
Chambersburg PA
CBHW080435290526
45791CB00008BA/2513